T0196220

Tales for Tagliacozzi

An Inside Look at Modern-Day Plastic Surgery

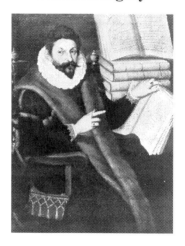

John Zannis, M.D.

authorHOUSE®

AuthorHouse™
1663 Liberty Drive
Bloomington, IN 47403
www.authorhouse.com
Phone: 1 (800) 839-8640

Published by AuthorHouse 01/09/2017

ISBN: 978-1-5246-5906-6 (sc)
ISBN: 978-1-5246-5907-3 (e)

Library of Congress Control Number: 2017900319

About the cover

Portrait of Gaspare Tagliacozzi ca. 1595 against the backdrop of Bologna, Italy, the home of Tagliacozzi and the world's oldest university.

Design by John Zannis, M.D.

Acknowledgements

Thank you to all of my professors at Wake Forest University for their instruction and patience during residency, especially Drs. Argenta and DeFranzo, who have a deep appreciation for the Renaissance Man.

Thank you to my parents who helped shape me.

Thank you to my amazing staff who keep the practice running.

Thank you to the editorial and production staff at Authorhouse Publishing.

A huge thank you to my wife, Stephanie, and our three precious children Gabriella, Alexander and Christopher. Without your love and endless support, none of it would be possible or worthwhile.

Finally, I thank God who gives me the strength.

Privacy Notice

All accounts in this book are based on true
patient interactions. Patient names have
been changed to protect their privacy.

All patients depicted in photographs have given
expressed written permission to publish their images.

Contents

About the Author

Plastic Surgery comes from the Greek word *plastikos*, meaning to shape, change or mold. It is the most creative and artistic field in medicine, and that is exactly what drew Dr. Zannis to this profession. Dr. Zannis grew up a scientist and an artist. He values a balance between his analytical left-brained personality and artistic right-brained sensibilities.

Studies in Florence, Italy instilled admiration for Leonardo and other Renaissance geniuses. Tagliacozzi, a surgical Renaissance genius, instilled artistry in the flesh. Much like Michelangelo's chisel freed the entrapped figures from blocks of Carrara marble, plastic surgeons all over the world strive to reveal their patients' true inner selves.

Dr. Zannis views his role as a problem-solver. "That's what plastic surgery is: a problem-solving specialty. It has been said that there is no specific boundary to the field. It is not limited to a certain body system the way cardiac surgeons only operate on the heart or urologists only treat the urinary system. Plastic surgery deals with all systems of the body from head to toe, including the skin, soft tissue, muscle and bone. It is more of an approach to surgical problems. How can a wound be healed? How can form and function be restored? How can rejuvenation be achieved?"

Dr. Zannis is an expert in face, breast and body procedures. Each patient is different and their concerns unique. "No two rhinoplasties are the same. Every facelift is its own distinct endeavor. That's what makes plastics so exciting. Every day is a challenge filled with interesting people and problems. The surgeries take precision and artistry, but the planning stage is what is really important. That's where all the work is." He values a natural-appearing result that maintains the individual's personality and unique characteristics.

Dr. Zannis is fluent in Greek, Italian & Spanish. His hobbies include carpentry, lutherie, and Mediterranean travel. He lives in New Bern, North Carolina with his wife and their three children. He is certified by the American Board of Plastic Surgery and directs a private practice and med-spa in New Bern.

Preface

Walking alone down Via dei Calzaiuoli, I felt eerily at home. The air in October was brisk and without all of the tourists, the streets were quieter. Florence like this felt more authentic. My daily walk through town and across the Arno to the Stanford Abroad campus was an opportunity for me to reflect on my time in Italy, my future, and all of the historic geniuses who had walked these roads before me. I am Greek, but I feel equally Italian. *Unna faccia, una razza.* One face, one race. I love art and Renaissance history. I love science and medicine. I love languages and travel. These are the things that drew me to Florence and the reason a part of my soul still resides there.

I marveled at the magnificent dome of Brunelleschi every day and the golden Baptistery doors that faced the duomo. I'd frequently trace my finger over a relief carving of a man's profile etched into the cornerstone of the Palazzo Vecchio. The carving was thought to be the work of Michelangelo. These innumerable reminders of the city's past connected me with their predecessors. I recall sipping an early morning espresso at my favorite café just the other side of the Old Bridge and wondering what it would have been like to live in the cinquecento – the golden century of the Italian Renaissance. I also contemplated where I would be in the future, say 10 years. Although I enjoyed art and architecture, I knew that for a career I was most interested in Medicine. I was certain that I would be a doctor. But, I had no idea that I would someday be a plastic surgeon.

Gaspare Tagliacozzi grew up in Bologna, Italy. A contemporary to Michelangelo and Leonardo, he would have walked similar cobblestone streets on his way to school. I'm sure he never imagined being a plastic surgeon either, let alone the founder of modern-day plastic surgery. First, he was a professor of surgery and anatomy, and later developed the so-called "Italian method" of plastic surgery in the mid-sixteenth century. I learned of Tagliacozzi as a surgical resident, primarily because his portrait is the symbol for the American Board of Plastic Surgery. As a resident, that's about all I had the time to learn regarding this Italian surgeon. But, as I matured in the field and gained more independence, I also gained more free time for reading. I actually purchased the definitive biography of Gaspare Tagliacozzi by Gnudi and Webster as well as a reprint of one of his most famous articles to learn more about one of Plastic Surgery's founding fathers.

Today, I spend my working days mostly at my private practice *The Zannis Center for Plastic Surgery* in New Bern, NC. I am the first to arrive, usually by 7am. I check my email and sort through charts left on my desk from the day before. Then, I review patient files and notes for the surgeries I am about to perform. Rhinoplasty, tummy tuck, and two breast augmentations. A great day. We steadily work through the cases, flip-flopping between two operating rooms, until 4pm. Then I reheat my cold coffee, make my operative reports and read more email. There are lots of bills to be paid, but I put that off usually until the next day.

Tagliacozzi performed rhinoplasties too. In fact, most say he invented rhinoplasty, or literally *shaping of the nose*. I'm sure his were different from the ones we do today. He hadn't discovered tip grafts or spreader grafts. I'm sure he would have been shocked to see what happened to Michael Jackson's infamous nose. I'm sure he would have been shocked by many things we do in the world of plastic surgery.

These thoughts are what led me to write this book. I hoped to reconnect with my Renaissance studies and rekindle my passion for Italian culture and history while delving more deeply into the life of my field's earliest forerunner. I wanted to share my delight as I imagined recounting the many unthinkable things that happen in my practice to someone like Gaspare Tagliacozzi. And, most importantly, I wanted to give a true insight into the life of a modern-day plastic surgeon. Prospective patients will learn a lot about the procedures available today. Everyone else will hopefully be amused.

Rhinoplasty

It is most fitting to begin with the nose. Rhinoplasty (*shaping of the nose*) is one of my favorite procedures. It is perhaps the most difficult procedure in plastic surgery and also one that has defined the specialty in the public's mind for many years. Rhinoplasty is also the procedure for which Gaspare Tagliacozzi is most famous. Most credit him with the invention of rhinoplasty itself.

It is difficult to say who invented a procedure that is so old and so varied in the ways it has been performed. Tagliacozzi, who lived from 1545 to 1599, was the first to explain in rational detail the principles of nose, lip and ear reconstruction. His *De Curtorum Chirurgia per Insitionem*, published in Venice in 1597, is considered the first book dedicated to plastic surgery. Many young plastic surgeons believe it was Rod who invented the specialty, but this is not true. Tagliacozzi (known by his friends as Tag) is the father of modern-day plastic surgery. But, Tag was preceded by a Hindu.

The plethora of Indian plastic surgeons is no accident. Susruta, as early as the 6th century BC, described in a basic text for Hindu medicine plastic methods for earlobe repair and nasal reconstruction. The nasal repair was performed by transposing a flap of skin from the cheek. Nose amputation was common in those days as a punishment for many crimes, and the repair therefore developed out of necessity.

Tagliacozzi has eloquently described his method for nasal reconstruction using brachial skin and subcutaneous fat in detail. He is akin to many modern plastic surgeons in his celebration of the art and his handiwork:

> Thus the art makes it possible to restore noses so satisfactorily that sometimes nature is surpassed, and if you except the color of the skin (which during the early days is not so healthy, yet there are means by which we improve it), you would not in any way detect the made nose, as anyone can testify by the evidence of his senses who has seen the noses restored by me this year. For there have been several gentlemen . . .of whom we restored noses so resembling nature's pattern, so perfect in every respect that it was their considered opinion that they liked these better than the original ones which they had received from nature.
>
> (From a letter to Hieronymus Mercurialis 1587)

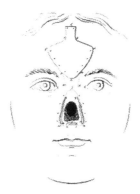

Diagram illustrating the median forehead flap known universally as the "Indian Method." (From Graefe, C.: Rhinoplastik, Berlin, Mit 6 Kupfertafeln, 1818.)

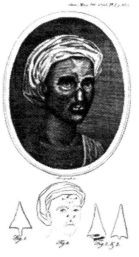

Illustration from the celebrated 1794 "Letter to Editor" responsible for the western spread of the "Indian Method" for total nasal reconstruction. (From B. L.: Letter to Editor. Gentlemans Magazine, October, 891, 1794.)

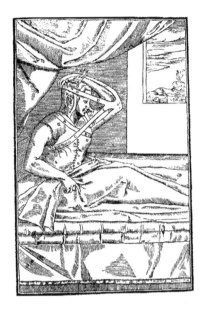

The "Italian Method"
(From Gnudi, M: The Life and Times of Gaspare
Tagliacozzi)

My rhinoplasty work certainly involves nasal reconstruction, not unlike the description of Tagliacozzi's procedure. It very common today to use forehead skin for a subtotal or total nasal reconstruction, like the "Indian Method." The tissue here is much more similar to the nose and it is more convenient for the patient to have a pedicled forehead flap than one from the arm (as the typical duration of attachment is 3 weeks).

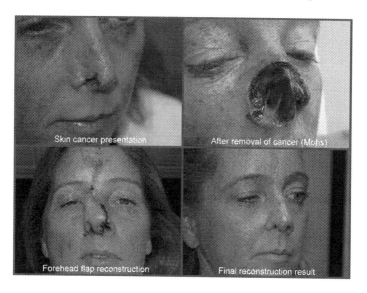

Skin cancer presentation

After removal of cancer (Mohs)

Forehead flap reconstruction

Final reconstruction result

One of my patients who presented with an advanced skin cancer of the nose.

However, today, rhinoplasty more typically refers to the cosmetic art of correcting a subjective nasal deformity. In other words, making someone's nose look nicer. Cosmetic rhinoplasty is something Tag would never have dreamt of as the surgeons of his era only treated deformities caused by trauma or disease. A purely cosmetic rhinoplasty is not even mentioned in history until the late nineteenth century.

Dr. John B. Roberts, in 1892, assured his colleagues that "nearly all undesirable distortions of the nose can be improved or entirely corrected by cosmetic operation ... the Roman nose, the Jewish nose, and the nose with an angular prominence on its dorsum can, in many instances, be satisfactorily modified." A great plastic surgeon once said that plastic surgery is restoring to normal what misfortune or disease has taken away. But where does cosmetic surgery fit in with this description? Subjective deformities are only deformities in the eyes of the beholder. Are we to fix what God made aesthetically displeasing to our current sensibilities? This philosophical discourse will be saved for another time.[1] But this is precisely what we do in rhinoplasty and all cosmetic procedures.

As a rhinoplasty specialist, I see many patients seeking this operation. What I tell them all is that I can do most anything to the nose. What is paramount is that I understand what you dislike and that we have perfect communication. There was a time in the eighties when excellent plastic surgeons were known for their trademark cookie cutter noses. It was a status symbol to have a "Sheen" nose or a "Gunter" nose. Fortunately, this is no longer in vogue. I talk to my patients about changing the displeasing attributes of the nose subtly to maintain one's unique characteristics and to fit harmoniously with the rest of the face. We are not all meant to have the same nose. As you can see, there truly is an art to rhinoplasty surgery, like most cosmetic surgery. The surgeon is entrusted to use his judgment and artistry during the procedure.

---

[1] I am a big supporter of cosmetic surgery if done for the right reasons and in the right setting. I have seen first-hand the effects such procedures can have on an individual's self-esteem and quality of life. The greatest challenge is determining who has the right motives and expectations. Surgical technique is usually much simpler than the complex psychology involved in this field.

The other component of a rhinoplasty is the airway. Our noses, of course, serve a purpose beyond mere beautification of the central aesthetic subunit of our face. The airway is actually a complicated series of valves and passageways whose alteration can be immediately recognized by the one breathing through it.

Some surgeons attempt to separate the two components — cosmetic and functional — but they truly are one organ that work in concert. You can really mess up someone's airway with just a cosmetic rhinoplasty if you aren't careful. The only thing angrier than a rhinoplasty patient who dislikes the appearance of their nose after surgery is one who suddenly can't breathe right after surgery.

I, like most responsible rhinoplasty surgeons, do a very detailed assessment of the airway to determine not only if I need to correct something while we're in there, but also how to avert problems.

I can only imagine sitting in Bologna's Estudia with Tag and exchanging accounts of our recent rhinoplasties. I'd tell him about dorsal humps and alar flaring. Hanging columellas and droopy tips. He'd look at me like I was a verified *pazzo* I'm sure. I'd tell him that attaching someone's arm to their face for a month was pretty crazy too.

I'd probably tell him about *Noah* too. He was an early rhinoplasty patient who has burned his story into my practice's collective memory, like many of the unique individuals you will hear about in this book. Noah was a 21 year-old Marine interested in reshaping his nose. Red flags: male rhinoplasty patient, young, slightly unrealistic about the expected ease of recovery and quick return to work. I did the procedure and it turned out very well. Of course, we did not let him drive to his hotel from the recovery room, as he planned. His vehicle remained in our parking lot for a few days because we sent him to the hotel with a friendly caregiver (nurse transport service). His recovery was uneventful, I assume, because he did not appear for any of his follow-up appointments until a year later. Only when he returned, it was under a new alias. He pretended he never met us and was here for an upper eyelid lift. I regretfully declined him for this procedure, not just because he was a little nuts, but because he didn't need it. The theory in our office was that he was in the process of transforming himself into a new person to further his career as an undercover spy.

Then there was *Juan Pablo*. Juan is my own personal Michael Jackson. A nice enough 39 year-old Hispanic patient who was seeking a "smaller" nose. Red flags: male rhinoplasty patient, Hispanic male patient, uses the word "smaller" to describe his rhinoplasty objective. Male rhinoplasty patients are very particular and very hard to please. Hispanic male patients are the most particular and difficult to please. It is my only patient population that makes it almost impossible to say no to repeat surgery. Juan underwent three revisions, continually striving for smaller. When he came in kindly pleading, "Por favor Doctor, una vez mas" just one more time? I had to say no. He almost cried at my denial, and I did feel sorry for him. I told him that his nose was going to disappear with *una vez mas*. He didn't find that very amusing. I assured him we were still friends and I cared for him, but I just could not do it. Sometimes, saying no is unquestionably the hardest thing to do.

The Procedure

The cosmetic rhinoplasty procedure can be done either open (through an incision in the columella at the base of the nose) or closed (through internal incisions only). If I plan to do any extensive tip work, then I choose the open approach. This allows complete visualization of the nose's cartilages.

After the patient is sedated and local anesthetic infiltrated into the nose, it is opened. This requires very meticulous technique to protect the fragile cartilages and thin skin around the nostrils. The plan, which is usually decided preoperatively based on the patient's anatomy and desires, is then executed systematically. This can include rasping of the dorsal hump, narrowing of the tip, excising cartilage from the lower lateral portions to refine the tip, and adding cartilage if needed for support or shape.

Cartilage grafts are very commonly used, and these are most often harvested from the septum. A cartilage graft can be used for many things including augmenting the dorsum, reshaping the tip, adding more projection to the tip or structurally reinforcing the ala (sides of the nose).

Finally, the airway is improved if not functioning properly. A deviated septum can be straightened and large turbinates (airflow regulators) can be reduced to allow for easier nasal respiration.

Once the nose is closed with sutures, external, and sometimes internal, nasal splints are applied. The patient is sent home from the recovery room with a drip pad and ice pack in place and returns to the office a week later for removal of the splints and sutures.

Average cost for rhinoplasty is $5,000-$6,000.

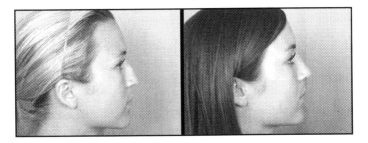

Patient of Dr. Zannis. Printed with permission.

Breast Augmentation

Two hills filled with snow and roses, with two little crowns of fine spouts at the top, like drinking straws for that beautiful and useful vessel. . . The breasts have a certain splendor, with such a novel charm, that we are forced to rest our eyes upon them in spite of ourselves.

- Agnolo Firenzuola, On the Beauty of Women

The Breast Implant

Vincenz Czerny has been called the "father of cosmetic breast surgery". In 1895 he published the first account of a breast implant which he had carried out, by moving a benign lipoma (fatty tumor) to "avoid asymmetry" after removing a cancerous tumor in a patient's breast.

A modern breast implant is a prosthesis used to change the size, form, and texture of a woman's breast. In plastic surgery, breast implants are used in post—mastectomy breast reconstruction, correcting congenital defects and deformities of the chest wall, and most notoriously for aesthetic breast augmentation.

There are two general types of breast implant devices today, defined by their filler material: saline solution or silicone gel. The saline implant has an elastomer silicone shell filled with sterile saline

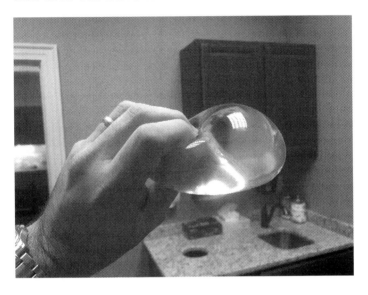

Example of modern silicone gel breast implants

solution; the silicone implant has an elastomer silicone shell filled with cohesive silicone gel. The latter implant has become the preferred device in my practice as well as internationally. Many refer to it as the "gummy bear" implant because it feels sort of like a gummy bear candy and maintains it shape the way a gummy bear would if it were cut in half. Hey Tag, nowadays we eat gummy bears and make larger versions to place in people's breasts. All kidding aside, they are very nice. Previous alternative composition implants featured miscellaneous fillers, such as soy oil and polypropylene string, and are no longer utilized in the United States.

Other discontinued breast implant filler substances include ivory, glass balls, ground rubber, ox cartilage, Terylene wool, gutta-percha, Dicora, polyethylene chips, Ivalon (polyvinyl alcohol—formaldehyde polymer sponge), a polyethylene sac with Ivalon, polyether foam sponge (Etheron), polyethylene tape (Polystan) strips wound into a ball, polyester (polyurethane foam sponge) Silastic rubber, and teflon-silicone prostheses. (Bondurant)

In 1961, two Houston plastic surgeons, Thomas Cronin and Frank Gerow, developed the first silicone breast implant with the Dow Corning Company. The following year, they performed the first modern-day breast implantation. Many generations of breast implants, including both silicone and inflatable saline varieties, have been produced since then. Since the mid-1990s, the fifth generation of silicone-gel breast implant has been made of a semi-solid gel that mostly eliminates the occurrences of filler leakage ("silicone-gel bleed") and of the migration of the silicone filler from the implant-pocket to elsewhere in the patient's body. An FDA moratorium on the use of silicone implants in the US from 1992-2005 was enforced to intensely research the effects of silicone implants on health. There was no evidence of systemic harm to the body found. In addition, the studies reported low incidence-rates of capsular contracture and of device-shell rupture; and greater medical safety than that of early generation breast implants.

The study *Effect of Breast Augmentation Mammoplasty on Self-Esteem and Sexuality: A Quantitative Analysis* (2007), reported that the women attributed their improved self-image, self-esteem, and increased, satisfactory sexual functioning to having undergone breast augmentation. The cohort, aged 21–57 years old, averaged post-operative self-esteem increases that ranged from 20.7 to 24.9 points on the 30-point Rosenberg self-esteem scale. Also, the data supported a 78.6 percent increase in the women's libido relative to pre-operative level of libido. (www. psychcentral.com)

There is no doubt that breast augmentation is a very gratifying procedure to perform. The effect it has on patients' self esteem and overall happiness is amazing. But, it is somewhat strange when viewed from an outsider's perspective. I recognized this when my eight-year-old daughter saw one of my medical journals and asked how the woman's breasts were made larger. I tried to evade the discussion, but her inquisitive mind wouldn't allow it. My rudimentary explanation was met with, "That's weird; you put a balloon under her skin to make her breasts bigger?" Yes it is a little weird. Lots of medicine is a little weird, though. I can only imagine Tagliacozzi having the same reaction my daughter had. "A balloon in the breast?!" Of course the procedure is more sophisticated than it appears. In fact, the intricacies of breast augmentation take years to learn and differentiate a great breast surgeon from an average one.

Along the way, I have augmented thousands of breasts. It is true that no two patients have the same breasts, *and no patient's two breasts are the same.* Preoperatively recognizing asymmetry as well as variances in anatomy is paramount to establishing a good operative plan. This is where experience is gained. My early results were unlikely as good as my latter results. I've learned how to spot important differences in breasts that as a novice surgeon I did not. The relationship of the inframammary fold to the nipple, the amount of skin stretch relative to the size of the breast, the propensity to experience a "double bubble" are all subtle factors that make a big difference in the end.

I've also learned how to identify a male seeking breast augmentation. Yes, I've been duped before. One memorable patient *Caprice*, saw me my first or second year in private practice for an augmentation. She was seeking to go from a small A cup to a C or D cup. She had a slender frame and was by all accounts a small-breasted woman who could really use my help to improve her identity as a woman. Well, that was an understatement. It wasn't until after her surgery, when my recovery nurse was helping her use the bathroom, that we discovered the truth about Caprice. It seems ridiculous to operate on someone without knowing his or her actual gender, but it wasn't the last time it happened. I personally do not perform transgender operations, so once in a while when we are asked about it, my staff says it is not something that I do. However, responding to the patient who claims to be a female in need of my help (though I or my staff have doubts about) is very challenging. How do you ask someone: "Are you really a man, because we can't do an augmentation on a man"? Imagine the hurt induced if the suspect patient was truly just an unfortunate woman.

My second (and I believe last) case of bamboozlement came the following year when *Jaime* came to see me. Jaime was a 6 foot tall husky lady with a deep voice and prominent Adam's apple. She already had implants placed many years ago, but one of the saline implants had leaked and she wanted a replacement. A little trickier scenario than that with Caprice. All signs pointed to a transgender patient. However, she was listed as female on her driver's license, had a husband, and had existing implants. She even told us that another surgeon had the audacity to refuse her an operation because he thought she was a man! Against the advice of my staff (a huge mistake) I acquiesced to Jaime. I couldn't ask for material proof — it would be too rude. I did, however, request that my recovery nurse confirm the situation while in the bathroom. Incredibly, she failed claiming, "If there was something there, it must have been well-tucked." I'd be too embarrassed even to attempt explaining "well-tucked" to our Italian friend Gaspare.

The Procedure

There are many variations in breast augmentation surgery. One variable is the operative approach, or incision placement. The implant can be inserted through the armpit, the nipple, or the crease beneath the breast. Some surgeons even attempt to place the breast implant through the belly button! This is not advised and actually voids the implant warranty if done. But the three other options are all viable. I have performed the three standard approaches and highly prefer the crease incision, also known as the inframammary fold (IMF) incision. The IMF incision has the best combination of ease of implant placement,

BREAST IMPLANT

Common placement options for breast implants

symmetry, and scar concealment. The armpit incision hides pretty well, but it is not good for consistently obtaining well-placed and symmetric implants. The nipple incision is not bad for placement, but has a more visible scar and a slightly higher risk for nipple sensitivity changes or difficulty with breast-feeding. Also, this route leads to capsular contracture, or hardening of the implant, more frequently.

So, I routinely will use the crease, or IMF incision. My patients are deeply sedated and the breast numbed with local anesthesia. After making the incision, the subpectoral muscle pocket is dissected. Placing the implant partly beneath the chest muscle has many advantages for the longevity of the implant, but it does take a little more work by the surgeon and causes more immediate soreness for the patient. Nevertheless, I explain the risk-benefit profile to all of my patients, and they agree that a week or two of a sore pec muscle is worth a more natural result with less long-term complications.

The "pocket" is then irrigated with antibiotic solution to avoid any risk of bacterial contamination. The implant is placed and then filled with saline if needed. Over 95% of the implants I place are silicone, and do not require the saline filling. Once final adjustments are made and the patient slightly sat up for inspection, the incision is closed and the same process is performed on the other side. The entire procedure takes approximately 45 minutes to perform. Patients go home the same day after recovering in the post-anesthesia area.

Average cost for breast augmentation is $5,000-$6,000.

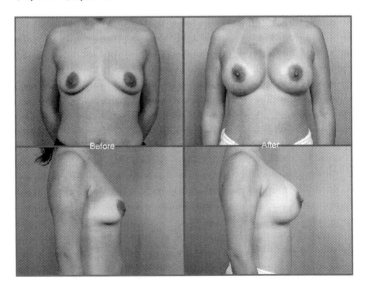

Patient of Dr. Zannis. Printed with permission.

Facelift

I wish I had a twin, so I could know what I'd look like without plastic surgery.

-Joan Rivers

Most cosmetic procedures seem to have the word "lift" appended to them. Breast lift, arm lift thigh lift, facelift, etc. Thanks to gravity (and the weakening of collagen and elastin in the skin with age), everything heads south as we get older. As a plastic surgeon, I am constantly fighting the forces of nature. To get lifted, in mind and body, is to restore youthful vitality. The facelift is a classic plastic surgery procedure, but it has not been around as long as many others.

A facelift, technically known as a rhytidectomy (from Ancient Greek ῥυτίς (rhytis) "wrinkle" + ἐκτομή (ektome) "excision", surgical removal of wrinkles), is a procedure used to give a more youthful facial appearance. There are multiple surgical techniques. It usually involves the removal of excess facial skin with tightening of underlying tissues, and the re-draping of the skin on the patient's face and neck.

From around 1900, surgeons began to play with the facial skin and excisional techniques that would tighten the skin of the face. This *cutaneous period* continued for nearly 70 years. In 1968, Dr. Skoog introduced the idea of subfascial dissection. This was the start of deeper tissue manipulation. Tessier, the Frenchman who had his background in craniofacial surgery, made the step to a subperiosteal dissection around 1980.

Today, most plastic surgeons have progressed to a technique that involves tightening of the SMAS, a thin muscle layer that supports the skin of the face, and some skin excision. More advanced techniques include a shorter scar length and some degree of volume restoration. The volume restoration attempts to replace, usually with fat, some of the facial fat which has been lost with age. I usually utilize a MACS lift, which stands for Minimal Access Cranial Suspension. This is a "real" facelift with a mini scar and less extensive dissection. This usually translates into a quicker surgery, a quicker recovery, and a more natural appearance. The overdone "windswept" look of bad Hollywood surgery is less than desirable.

The ability to recognize oneself even after a second facelift is very desirable. One of the greatest fears patients have when considering a facelift is coming out looking weird or unrecognizable. I fully appreciate that fear and begin by telling my patients that my goal is to help them look and feel younger and better, but still like themselves. I want everyone they meet to compliment them, but not know that they've had anything done.

Nevertheless, some people go out and tell everyone that they've had something done. They're proud of themselves and want others to notice. One such patient of mine was *Rafaella*, an Italian immigrant who had a facelift in her late sixties. She was a self-described "cougar" who had her sights fixed on 30-year old men. She was charming and naturally beautiful, but she had the sagging skin of a 60-year old lady. This did not provide her with the competitive edge she desired, and she didn't look the way she felt inside.

I got a little bit stressed out when she was going to sleep for surgery and started mumbling things about *Dio* and *Cielo*, God and Heaven. Tagliacozzi would be happy to hear that his compatriot did very well during surgery and awoke just fine. She was admittedly confused for a few minutes and the first thing she said to me in the recovery room was, "Are you God?" Not a great thing to hear from any patient! No, it's just me — Dr. Zannis.

The Procedure

I remember the first time I participated in a facelift. I was assisting Dr. DeFranzo (i.e. watching him do his magic). I was truly amazed by the complexity of the case, yet simplicity of the tailoring. He trimmed off excess skin, and tacked part of it up. Then trimmed off some more, and tightened a little more. Slowly, the patients face took shape the way a hand-made Italian suit is custom tailored. I fell in love with this procedure at that moment.

Although skin is usually removed and tightened, the most important element of a facelift is the re-suspension of the SMAS muscle mentioned earlier. Access to this layer of muscle begins with the incision. After local anesthetic is injected into the subcutaneous layers of the face and neck, the incision is made. I usually begin in the temporal hair, continue down just in front of the ear in a natural crease found there, and around the bottom of the earlobe to the crease behind the ear. This incision heals and hides remarkably well. From here, the skin flap is elevated just enough to expose the underlying structures that are manipulated. Occasionally fat is removed. The muscle is then tightened by lifting it and securing it to a higher position with permanent sutures. This is the step that keeps the lifted result intact for many years. Excess skin is then trimmed with DeFranzoesque finesse. And then, everything is closed up.

An important concept in a facelift, as well as most other surgeries, is hemostasis. Hemostasis means no bleeding. The operative field is dry and there is little risk of bleeding after the closure and formation of a clot of blood under the skin called a hematoma. This kind of blood clot won't hurt you, but if undiagnosed, it can hurt the overlying skin and sometimes lead to a wound. For this reason, all facelift patients must be evaluated the day after surgery.

I like to wrap the face with a cold compression dressing to help minimize swelling and promote healing in the newly lifted state. Patients wear this wrap for a week. Biggest complaint after a facelift: can't wash your hair for a couple of days!

Average cost for facelift is $7,000-$10,000.

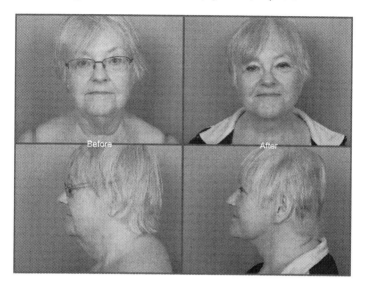

Patient of Dr. Zannis. Printed with permission.

Abdominoplasty

The tummy tuck. It is such an amazing euphemism for a relatively intense procedure. Plastic surgeons definitely have a way to make procedures sound better than they should. Everything we do is either lift or tuck. This is our first tuck procedure to be discussed. And, there is also the cute little sister to the tummy tuck, the *mini* tummy tuck.

Abdominoplasty began in the late 1800s when a surgeon named Kelly removed the extra midsection of a patient. The scar was horrible, and the procedure very far from the artistic tummy tucks of today, but it solved a problem. In the 1970s, the bikini line incision became popular as the entire scar could be hidden while wearing a 2 piece bathing suit. Interestingly, the bikini's cut has changed over the years (high cut, low cut, French cut, etc.), and this has necessitated the adaptation of the plastic surgeon's scar placement. Today, low bikinis are in vogue and it is not uncommon for patients to request their incision be placed very close to the neverlands region. Of course, we learned in residency that you must leave at least 3-4 cm from this area or you risk distorting the vulva.

When it comes to the results from a tummy tuck, it is fair to say that you see better outcomes in patients who are in better shape. In other words, the lower the BMI (Body Mass Index), the better the result. This is often an applicable generalization for many different procedures. In the case of abdominoplasty, if there is less fat to remove and mostly loose, excess skin to contend with, the shape turns out nicer. Also, there is less risk for complications like seroma, infection, and DVT, or blood clots.

Unfortunately, the majority of patients seeking tummy tucks are not ideal candidates. Not to say that they don't benefit immensely from the surgery, but that they are at slightly higher risk for problems and they are less likely to have an amazing result. In addition, performing a tummy tuck in an obese patient is significantly more difficult and tiring for the surgeon. As it is with everything in surgery, you must use your best judgement in evaluating these patients and counseling them. I don't offer surgery to every patient. But, they sure do make it hard for you to say no. As long as the benefits outweigh the risks and there is a clear understanding of what to expect as a result (i.e. realistic expectations), I will agree to the surgery.

"Who approved this?" is a question I posed many years ago upon entering a tummy tuck case and viewing the patient on the table. It has become a comical phrase around my office because it seems as if it applies to half of my cases. Obesity is clearly a huge problem in our society. As a plastic surgeon, the sequelae of obesity, both physical and emotional, are an integral part of my practice. But, weight loss surgery is not a part of plastic surgery. That is bariatric surgery, and patients should not expect to lose much weight from a body contouring procedure. I always say it's about the inches in plastic surgery, not the pounds.

There is a related procedure to the tummy tuck called a panniculectomy. This means removal of the abdominal pannus, or large apron of skin and fat hanging from a patient's belly. Sometimes, insurance companies will pay for a panniculectomy because it has medical implications, not just cosmetic. The pannus can get infected and ulcerated. The rash beneath it can be very painful and nearly impossible to control with topical medications. However, insurance companies are not too fond of covering these procedures any more. The problem is that too many people sought tummy tucks under the guise of a panniculectomy. I still have patients calling every week seeking a tummy tuck paid for by insurance. It doesn't work, and we don't even try. Unless there are chronic, non-healing wounds on the pannus, I consider it a cosmetic procedure and the patient is responsible for payment out-of-pocket.

The belly button is an interesting feature of the human torso. After birth, the belly button, or umbilicus, serves no purpose. Yet, a lot of care goes into recreating an aesthetically pleasing belly button during a tummy tuck. It is very true that our eye appreciates a properly shaped and properly placed belly button. Sometimes with a panniculectomy, the belly button is sacrificed. And, although most of these patients accept that fine, some will respond as if it is a great tragedy to lose this stretched out piece of invaginated abdominal skin. The other thing about tummy tucks and the belly button is the wide assortment of stuff you find in a belly button.

My nurses prep the patients before surgery with antiseptic cleaning solution, and the belly button must be cleaned out too. One of my nurses has a proclivity to vomiting when there is anything retrieved from the patient's belly button. What has been retrieved? Well, there's the usual navel fuzz, dirt, food crumbs, and one time we found a tooth. Yes, it looked and smelled like a rotten tooth. I'm sure it was just calcified cheesy skin exudate which had been impacted in the unexplored umbilicus for years, but it sounds cooler to say, "I found a tooth in her belly button!"

The Procedure

My abdominoplasties always start with liposuction. You mustn't underestimate the importance of liposuction during a tummy tuck because the hourglass waistline frequently can't be achieved without aggressive liposuctioning. It is taught that aggressive liposuctioning, especially in the central abdomen, is risky during a tummy tuck. However, if you know what you're doing, it's not a problem at all. After infiltrating with tumescent solution (which we'll discuss in the next chapter) and waiting for a few minutes so it takes effect, I liposuction. The flanks/"love handles" and anterior abdomen are thoroughly liposuctioned. Sometimes the mons needs to be suctioned too. The mons pubis is the pubic mound that often looks very exaggerated after a tummy tuck is completed in a large patient. In my early days, patients would ask me why I made their mons bigger. I would accurately respond, "I didn't. It was always that big; it's just that now you can see it." They understood, but didn't feel much better. So now, I lipo all of the big monses, or *mons*ters.

The next step is the dissection, where usually a low bikini incision is made and the skin flap elevated off of the anterior abdominal wall. The belly button must be incised and freed so that the dissection can continue up to the sternum. Along the way, perforating blood vessels are cauterized and then we keep going in search of the xyphoid process (the little bony protrusion at the bottom of the sternum). I think I'm on a road trip with my kids when I hear, "Are we there yet?" But it is only my surgical tech implying that her arm is getting tired of retracting.

After the dissection, I normally plicate the rectus muscle fascia. This is referred to as "tightening the muscles" because most patients have a separation of their abdominal muscles and a weakness that causes a noticeable bulge in the belly. This muscle tightening, in my opinion, is one of the most important, yet underappreciated, steps of the abdominoplasty procedure. It is also the part of the procedure which leads to the majority of pain afterwards.

Next, the excess skin is resected while sitting the patient in a beach chair position to maximize the amount of skin that can be removed. The incision is closed over two percutaneous drainage tubes. We also have a few newer techniques that can be used instead of placing drainage tubes.

Usually 2-3 lbs of tissue are resected. Finally, the belly button is recreated and sutured into place looking as pretty as possible. Dressings are placed and an abdominal compression binder is fitted prior to the patient waking up from anesthesia.

Average cost for abdominoplasty is $7,000-$9,000.

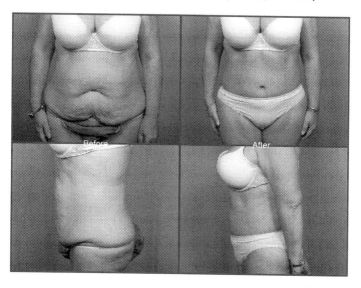

Patient of Dr. Zannis. Printed with permission.

Liposuction

Liposuction is one of those quintessential plastic surgery procedures that most lay people are somewhat familiar with. It is remarkably barbaric in concept (and sometimes appearance) yet quite dependent on finesse and artistry to achieve a nice cosmetic result. The idea is basic: insert a tube into the body through a small hole to suck out unwanted fat. I sometimes wonder how such a simple idea could be made so complicated (ex. SlimLipo™, SmartLipo™, Vaser™, SafeLipo™). One liposuction textbook by Shiffman and DiGiuseppe is 948 pages long!

In fact, liposuction, or suction assisted lipectomy, is little more than sucking out fat with a vacuum. The invention of the modern liposuction procedure is attributed to two of Tagliacozzi's compatriots, Italian physicians Arpad and Giorgio Fischer. They created the blunt tunneling method in 1974. Then, liposuction gained tremendous attention due to a presentation by the French surgeon Dr. Yves-Gerard Illouz in 1982. The "Illouz Method" featured a technique of suction-assisted lipolysis after infusing fluid into tissues using blunt cannulas (tumescent) and high-vacuum suction and demonstrated both reproducible good results and low complications, or morbidity. Another French surgeon, Pierre Fournier used lidocaine as local anesthetic, and began to use compression after the operation to minimize postoperative swelling.

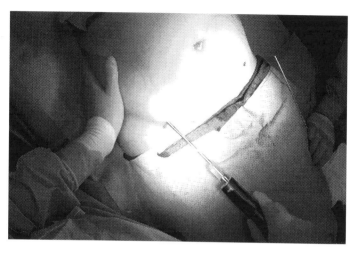

An intraoperative photo of me performing Power Assisted Liposuction

During the 1980s, many American surgeons experimented with liposuction, developing various forms of sedation techniques to avoid general anesthesia, as well as using a "superwet" tumescent technique to minimize blood loss and further improve the safety of the procedure. As long as candidates are selected appropriately, a qualified surgeon performs the procedure, and the setting is an accredited surgical facility, liposuction should be very safe and reproducible.

As physicians and scientists tend to do, we complicate simple concepts in an attempt to "improve" them. In many ways, liposuction techniques have improved tremendously. And, although the introduction of ultrasound and laser assistance has contributed to the abilities of the modality, liposuction has always been about one thing: sucking out the fat.

A patient that I will never forget had the staged procedure called *lipo-abdo-umbo*. Casey, a young Marine, had a waist problem. If you can't make weight in the Marine Corps, they use an archaic measurement system where a ratio of your neck circumference and waist circumference (measured at the level of the umbilicus) determines if you are fit enough to serve our country. Casey was decidedly unfit due to his waistline. If he did not remedy this problem within a few months, he would be discharged from the Marine Corps and be out of a job and the benefits his family needed. So, like many other young servicemen in his predicament, he came to see me for help.

We talked through the options and elected to proceed with liposuction, which ended up reducing his waist by 2 inches – not enough. We figured his redundant skin had to go because it contributed excess tissue that liposuction could not address. So, we next proceeded to the abdominoplasty. This was great and his abdomen looked awesome – not enough! What was the problem? Well, it turns out that Casey had a low umbilicus (belly button). The required measurements are taken at the level of the belly button, where in Casey's case the hips were contributing unnecessarily to his measurement. We came up with a plan to save Casey's career: move the umbo. Yes, move the umbilicus to a higher position on the abdomen where his waist was naturally (and after 2 surgeries) much narrower. To this day, Casey continues to have one of the best-looking, and most interesting, abdomens in the Marine Corps.

The Procedure

Vaser™ is an ultrasound-assisted liposuction technique that I utilized as a resident. Its main benefit over traditional methods was the emulsification of the fat, which allowed for less traumatic extraction, and skin tightening due to the thermal energy produced by the ultrasound. The problem with it was sometimes the skin would get burned and it was more tedious and took longer to do. I used SmartLipo™ for many years too. This was an improvement over Vaser™ because it used a small fiberoptic laser cannula to melt the fat and also tighten the skin, but with more ease and less risk for skin burning. However, it was more expensive and also time-consuming. Now days, I primarily use a technique called Safelipo™. Safelipo™ uses no ultrasounds, lasers, or other expensive machines. It is a more pure return to traditional superwet liposuction. However, the cannula tips and the physical method of performing it, allow for smoother contours with much less dents or other irregularities that have always plagued liposuction.

Liposuction can be performed on most areas of the body, including the face, neck arms and most commonly abdomen, flanks, back and thighs. I perform the procedure under IV sedation with the patient spontaneously breathing. It can be done with just local anesthesia (or tumescent), but most patients find this to be uncomfortable, especially when large areas are being treated. As the tissue expands

33

under the pressure of the tumescent fluid (which comes from the Latin word *tumor*, meaning swelling) an awake patient can experience significant pain. So, we choose to do this asleep.

Next, an assortment of liposuction cannulas, or tubes, are used to suction the unwanted fat from the areas of concern. I love doing this with the power-assisted hand piece which vibrates in a fashion that breaks up the fat and removes it more easily and smoothly.

When the desired contour is achieved, excess fluid is removed from the tissue and then compression garments are placed to help reduce post-operative swelling. The final results are visible after 2-3 months.

Average cost for liposuction is $4,000-$6,000.

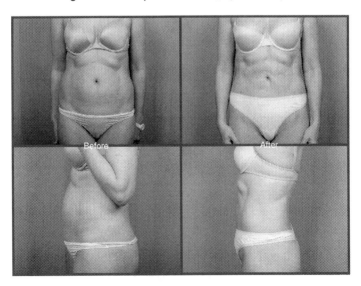

Patient of Dr. Zannis. Printed with permission.

Periorbital Rejuvenation

The eyes are the windows to the soul and the subject of art, poetry and plastic surgery alike. The history of eyelid surgery dates back to approximately 25 A.D. when a roman philosopher named Aulus Cornelius Celsus described the excision of upper eyelid skin for the "relaxed eyelid" in his *De Re Medica*. It is unclear whether he was describing an eyelid ptosis or an excess of skin. In 1818, Von Graefe first used the term 'blepharoplasty" to describe a case of eyelid reconstruction following a cancer resection. Many European surgeons began discussing the blepharoplasty procedure to correct functional eyelid problems around this time.

In the early 1900's, many surgeons began to popularize the removal of upper eyelid skin for aesthetic enhancement. In 1907, the American Conrad Miller wrote one of the first books on cosmetic surgery, *Cosmetic Surgery in the Correction of Facial Imperfection*, in which he diagrammed blepharoplasty incisions very similar to the ones used today.

Since then, many advancements have occurred, including lower blepharoplasty, trans-conjunctival approaches (incisions from inside the eyelid), removal of fat from bulging lids, and precise closure techniques. In addition, the importance of thorough preoperative evaluation, identification of dry eyes and other ocular symptoms have been well-described.

I personally love the blepharoplasty procedures, particularly the upper. The reason is because it is a straight-forward and safe operation that instantly rejuvenates the face with little discomfort or downtime for the patient. Friends and family of the patient universally find them more refreshed, youthful and healthy looking, without being able to pinpoint the reason why (i.e. others will know you look good without knowing you've had a procedure!).

Javier knew particularly well how important the eyes were to the overall aesthetic of a person's face. He was a 50 year old Mexican immigrant who had deep facial wrinkles and badly sun-damaged skin. None of that bothered him. What bothered him most was his excess upper eyelid skin. It didn't affect his vision, but it felt "heavy and looked horrible."

I performed an upper blepharoplasty for Javier. A few months later, I performed a second one on his right side. A few months after that he had a brow lift to get the brows and lids pulled even higher. He ended up looking quite good, and not overdone. But, I just couldn't understand his motivation for this. He would not stop until it was just how he wanted. Once again, I never knew the Hispanic male would be one of the most persistent and demanding cosmetic surgery patients.

The Procedure

An upper blepharoplasty can be performed with local anesthesia or sedation. The lower lids usually are best done under sedation. After markings are made to confirm how much skin should be removed, yet still ensure the eye can close, the lids are anesthetized with local anesthesia. I always wait 7 minutes to ensure the epinephrine has had enough time to effectively cause vasoconstriction for minimal bleeding.

After the skin is excised, a small strip of muscle and then bulging pockets of fat can be removed. The goal is to eliminate puffiness without creating a hollowed out or sunken look. After meticulous care to stop all bleeding, the incision is closed with a single suture in a running fashion under the surface of the skin.

Patients experience some bruising and swelling, and maybe a little dry eye for a week or so. Pain is minimal and rarely are pain meds needed. At one month, the final result is appreciated and scars are imperceptible.

Average cost for upper blepharoplasty is $2,500-$3,500.

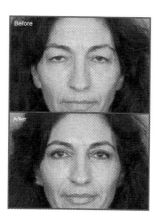

Patient of Dr. Zannis. Printed with permission.

Butt Lift

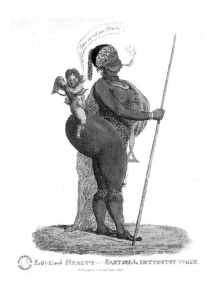

Hottentot Venus

The Hottentots were a Southwest African race whose descendants today are called Khoikhoi. The Dutch settlers of the mid-17th century named them "Hottentots" after the clicking language they spoke.

Two of the females' distinct physical attributes were very long genital labia and extremely large buttocks. In fact, many early images show women whose derrieres came off at a right angle from the lower back. To the men of that culture, this was considered a beautiful figure and sign of health and good childbearing capabilities (although the long labia were usually trimmed prior to marriage).

Today, we've seen a revival of the Hottentot standard of beauty. In fact, you could almost consider Kim Kardashian a descendant of the Hottentots (or Hotties for short). Kim Kardashian most likely had some buttock augmentation to achieve her Hottie appearance, although she has publicly denied this in the past.

Si, Signore Tagliacozzi . . . vogliano un culo grandissimo. Tagliacozzi would never understand why women today would want a huge butt. Almost daily, my office is contacted by a patient seeking the now famous Brazilian Butt Lift. A procedure named after the country that popularized it, the BBL involves suctioning fat from unwanted areas of the body, straining it, and then injecting it into the buttocks. The goal is a large, round butt a *la* Jennifer Lopez or Kim K.

For some reason, this turns out to be the most unreliable patient population. It has nothing to do with race, culture, or socioeconomic status. Whatever the reason may be, butt lift patients are notorious for not showing up to their appointments. It got so bad that we began collecting the consult fee by credit card over the phone if you wanted to reserve a BBL initial consult appointment.

The other problem with the Brazilian Butt Lift procedure is there's never enough fat. At least, there's never enough to please some patients. Some people want really huge butts, and there is not enough fat in there body to put in the butt. I really want my patients to be completely thrilled with their cosmetic results, but I also feel a responsibility as the physician "artist" to impose some of my aesthetic sensibilities into the case. I am up front with prospective candidates for surgery and tell them what I think I can achieve, what I would like to achieve and my personal approach. I try to fuse this with their desires so we are both happy with the results.

The Procedure

The Brazilian Butt Lift procedure is simply a fat transfer procedure. It involves harvesting fat from unwanted areas of the body via liposuction and then injecting it into the buttocks. The harvesting part and contouring of the torso, has a lot to do with the final result. Removing fat from the waist and lower back instantly improves the appearance of the buttocks.

Then, the patient's harvested fat is strained, or washed and prepared into syringes for transfer. There are hundreds of methods and surgical contraptions marketed for doing this part. I first began with a stainless steel kitchen strainer and spoon (that was cleaned and sterilized before reuse) to fill my syringes. My surgical tech at the time referred to it as "cooking," and she really enjoyed it. It made a huge mess with slippery fat grease all over the floor and "tomato basil soup" all over the walls. Not the most elegant method, but it worked.

My BBL technique has evolved to a much neater and streamlined process today. We use professionally-made suction canisters with internal strainers made solely for the purpose of fat harvesting. No one slips and slides anymore, and although we sometimes miss cooking, this system is quite a bit more efficient.

After the fat is injected into the proper planes and a nice, full, symmetric buttock is achieved, we close up and place the patient in a compression garment. He or she must not place excessive pressure on the buttocks for a couple weeks. This means no long periods of sitting or sleeping on your back during early recovery. After that, the transposed fat has taken permanent residence in its new home where it lives happily ever after.

Average cost for Brazilian Butt Lift is $5,000-$7,000.

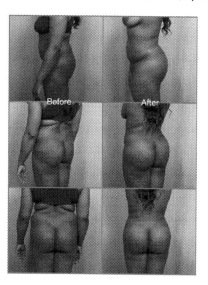

Patient of Dr. Zannis. Printed with permission.

41

Smoking

Giving up smoking is the easiest thing in the world. I know because I've done it a thousand times.

-Mark Twain

Smoking is a strange phenomenon with a long history in human society. Although Gaspare Tagliacozzi might not have been introduced to tobacco (it was brought to France by the Frenchman Jean Nicot in 1560), he was surely familiar with the practice of smoking.

Smoking various mind-altering or hallucinogenic substances had been done for thousands of years. In ancient India, China and the Middle East, opium and cannabis were smoked through pipes for religious rituals and eventually for pleasure. Since early in Christian rituals, Greek Orthodox Christians burned incense during their services, not to get high, but because of the way the smell and sometimes the inhaled chemicals helped put them in proper mood for worship.

Over the past 60 years, we have discovered the many detrimental effects of habitual nicotine use. It's bad for your lungs, your cardiovascular system, and can lead to cancer. Smoking and its ill effects are of particular concern to plastic surgeons, perhaps more than any other type of surgeon. Tagliacozzi would have been intrigued to learn that the substance people intentionally inhale for pleasure or habit, has profound effects on wound healing. Certain procedures like facelifts and tummy tucks could end up in disaster if performed on an active smoker.

Nicotine constricts blood vessels, and a few small blood vessels are all the skin of some flaps (or sections of skin and soft tissue) in plastic surgery procedures depend on for life-giving oxygen. Constrict too many of those little vessels, and your skin flaps can die. I've seen it many times, usually in patients who lie about not smoking or those in which an urgent procedure is needed and we can't afford to wait for them to quit smoking for 6 weeks before surgery.

I performed a breast reduction on a patient named Kelly who was an active smoker. We discussed all of the risks involved with smoking prior to surgery and the need for her to quit smoking before we could proceed with the reduction. Some procedures, for example liposuction, are not exceedingly riskier to smokers. Others like breast reductions or facelifts and tummy tucks as already mentioned, are significantly riskier. She quit smoking for 6 weeks prior to surgery, which studies have shown is the amount of time needed for your microvasculature to "return to normal" after smoking cessation.

Things went well with Kelly for a week or so before we began to notice problems. A lot of the skin edges near her incisions on the right breast began turning dusky and eventually black. A lot of the skin died, and she also suffered fat necrosis, or death, in that breast which required two surgical debridements before we were left with tissue healthy enough to heal itself. For unexplainable reasons, the left side healed fine.

Why did this happen? It was quite clear to me and my staff that Kelly had resumed smoking right after her surgery (or maybe even never fully quit). She reeked of smoke at every post-op visit and blamed it on her chain-smoking mother who rode with her to the visits. Second-hand smoking is bad enough to have caused her complications, but my hunch is there was some first-hand smoking involved as well.

Another patient named *Cindy* was a boisterous Vietnamese lady who had been saving for a tummy tuck for years. In fact, she stopped by my office and made payments towards the procedure for many months until it was all paid up. The problem was her smoking and the fact that she had not yet quit as we had planned. I warned her that I would be administering a urine nicotine test on the day of her pre-op history and physical exam and she would not be able to fool us.

Well, Cindy showed up for her pre-op visit and when it came time for the urine test, she asked one of my nurses if she would pee in the cup for her! She actually expected one of my employees to play accomplice in her attempt at urine nicotine testing fraud! Of course my nurse declined, and Cindy was refunded all of her money. We found out a few weeks later from a coworker of hers that she had gone to Mexico for her tummy tuck and was now having some sort of "problems."

I don't judge those who smoke. Actually, I am a big fan of cigars and find value in the relaxation they offer. I justify cigar smoking by the fact that I don't inhale the smoke. And, it is true that cigars smoked occasionally are less threatening than cigarettes smoked regularly. Like everything else, it's up to each individual to choose what he or she does with their bodies. But, when it comes to smoking and plastic surgery, the two are often mutually exclusive. And, this applies to all nicotine sources including gum, patches and e-cigarettes.

The Recovery Room

You might be a PACU nurse if....

You're shopping in the store and warn the
loaf of bread in the cart that there's a bump
coming.

The PACU, or *Post Anesthesia Care Unit*, is where patients
go immediately after their procedure is completed. Here,
they recover from anesthesia and slowly wake up and
resume a near normal level of consciousness before being
discharged to home with their caretaker.

We prefer to use what is called MAC anesthesia, which
stands for Monitored Anesthesia Care. In other words, the
patients are sedated and generally unconscious, but are
breathing without the assistance of a ventilator. This differs
from General Anesthesia where inhalational gases are
normally used and the patient is placed on a ventilator via
a breathing tube for the duration of the case.

The reason I love a deep MAC anesthetic is because
it usually provides an easier recovery from the patient's
perspective: less nausea or vomiting, no sore throat from

the endotracheal tube, and less grogginess. These are all positives when performing outpatient surgery. The trick is it takes an anesthetist with exceptional skills to balance the level of sedation safely and appropriately to the surgeon's needs. We are fortunate to have Bob, the best CRNA in North Carolina, and his team of experts provide our anesthesia. When Bob is done waking them up, patients proceed to the adjacent PACU for transition of care to a recovery nurse.

The PACU is a fun and interesting place sometimes. Patients emerging from anesthesia often show an uninhibited side of themselves that is clearly drug-induced. Think of an introverted friend who's had a few too many drinks. A lot of the drugs used, like propofol, can be considered truth serums. When patients are going to sleep or waking up from their anesthetic, an uninhibited string of gibberish often occurs.

It's funny when they say stuff that you'd never expect. We talked about Noah earlier. He woke up mumbling about Lindsay Lohan and how he wanted to go out partying with her in Vegas. I also mentioned Rafaella's sincere, yet frightening, inquiry: "Are you God?" I was fortunate enough to perform a few different surgeries for a patient named Kary. She went to sleep and woke up every time talking about what the stripper name would be for my various staff members. It was quite entertaining, and she was always jovial and never irritating.

One of the most memorable cases was *Narnia*. She was a Middle Eastern patient who spoke good, but accented

English. She woke up wild — swinging and punching at everyone in sight. She didn't' want anything to do with the crackers we offered her spitting them out at my nurse while exclaiming, "These crackers are cheap! You need to buy higher quality snacks for your patients." It was slightly offensive, but also hard to resist laughing at that moment. Things got awkward when she started spewing epithets about her husband who was waiting just outside the door. "He's a horrible husband. I hate him." *Okay, Narnia . . . I think it's time to go now.*

Secrets

I'd like to begin the conclusion of this book by stating how much I love my job and how truly honored I am to have so many people place their trust in me. I can't imagine a more rewarding profession. This is why I have decided to reveal some insider information, or trade secrets about cosmetic surgery practice today. Many in the field would argue that this should not be revealed to the public. However, I feel a strong moral obligation to be honest and fully transparent with my patients and prospective patients. It is only with clear and factual information that patients can make informed decisions that are good for themselves and their loved ones. I frame these secrets in the context of 5 questions you must ask your plastic surgeon before having surgery, and then conclude with 5 highly classified secrets.

The 5 Most Important Questions You Must Ask Your (Plastic) Surgeon Before Having Surgery

1. Are you certified by the American Board of Plastic Surgery?

This is probably the most important question. The American Board of Plastic Surgery certifies surgeons who have successfully completed a residency training program in Plastic Surgery. You must prove safety and competency by undergoing a very vigorous written and oral exam process. 20-30% of eligible applicants fail each year, so it is **NOT** an easy thing to accomplish. Are there good surgeons out there who trained in plastic surgery but did not obtain their board certification? Absolutely. However, it is hard to sort them out and board certification at least gives you a starting point, or basic level of confidence, that your surgeon is well-qualified.

And, don't be fooled by illegitimate "board certifications." There are only select boards that are officially recognized by the American Board of Medical Specialties. In plastic surgery, the only recognized board is the American Board of Plastic Surgery.

Most board certified plastic surgeons also belong to the American Society for Plastic Surgeons, and their logo looks like this:

Member

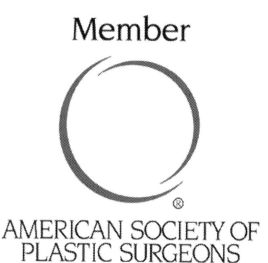

AMERICAN SOCIETY OF PLASTIC SURGEONS

A sensitive topic: For many years now, the reimbursement for physician services has been declining. Couple that with increasing physician regulations and piles of insurance-related paperwork, and doctors are more frustrated than ever. This has led many non-plastic surgeons to venture into the field of cosmetic medicine. This is an enormous problem and a world-wide phenomenon, though worst in the U.S. It is not unusual to find family doctors, anesthesiologists, oral surgeons and dentists, and many more, performing botox®, facial fillers, dermabrasion, etc. Now there are "non-core" physicians performing surgery too. In my average-sized town, there are radiologists performing liposuction, ENT doctors doing breast augmentation and eye doctors doing facelifts! This is irresponsible and unsafe, but totally legal. A doctor can practice any type of medicine he or she chooses, even without specialty training in that field.

Would you want an unqualified doctor performing your surgery? Of course not! But patients are usually not educated enough to recognize the situation, and the non-plastic surgeons posing as plastic surgeons are certainly not going to voluntarily offer up that information. Even if asked, "Are you a plastic surgeon," or "Are you board-certified," they are likely to provide an ambiguous, less-than-truthful response. "I have been performing cosmetic procedures for many years" or "I am a board certified doctor" are common, yet dubious answers. Board certified in what? Board certification in obstetrics and gynecology does not qualify you to perform a tummy tuck or liposuction just because the patient is a woman!

I am ashamed to admit that there such charlatans among us in the medical profession, but it is the honest truth. Usually the search for an easy buck comes back to bite these doctors because making the buck is not that easy. It takes a lot of hard work and training to learn how to be a real cosmetic surgeon, and it is still hard work after that. The unfortunate thing is that many patients suffer along the way.

2. Do you specialize in this area / procedure?

As a plastic surgeon, I was trained in all areas of the field including, cosmetic surgery, reconstructive surgery, facial trauma, hand surgery and congenital deformities. However, there are certain procedures that I never performed again once I left my training program. For example, I haven't performed a cleft lip repair since I was a chief resident, but I perform nearly 10 breast augmentations every week. Likewise, a pediatric plastic surgeon may perform cleft lip repairs weekly, but never do breast implants. The point is that you want your surgery to be done by someone who performs that procedure very frequently and has a mastery of the subtle nuances that come with any procedure. **You want a specialist.** I specialize in facial cosmetic surgery, breast surgery and tummy tucks. I also perform other procedures, like the Brazilian Butt Lift, once or twice a month. I feel very capable with those procedures and think I am safe and do a good job. But I would not claim to be an international authority or specialist, and I inform every patient of the fact that I specialize in certain procedures like breast augmentation and not in others.

How can you recognize a specialist? This is not usually that difficult to do. First, you ask around town, ask your friends, ask other doctors. Who is recommended for certain types of procedures? You can search the internet and look for reviews. Just because someone declares themselves a specialist, doesn't mean they are one. If the popular and professional consensus is that they are, then they probably are.

Have they had additional training in a subfield of plastic surgery? Examples would include a fellowship in hand or microsurgery, or a fellowship in craniofacial surgery. These fellowships indicate an extra commitment and higher level of understanding of that particular area.

The easiest way to determine if your doctor is a specialist is to look at their before and after pictures. If they don't freely offer before and after pictures on their website, be very skeptical. This is the standard expectation, and an absence of a photo gallery usually means either their work is less than stellar, or they have very few patients and results to show. Inspect the quality of their results, but also look for the number of photos. As I've said before, one of the things I specialize in is breast enhancement, and I have hundreds of breast patients in my photo gallery. Likewise, someone who specializes in facelifts should have hundreds of facelift photos to show, not just two or three.

3. What results can I realistically expect?

Everyone hopes for a great result — both the surgeon and patient. Nevertheless, everyone doesn't get a great result. Sometimes this is completely unforeseen, but often it is predictable. I know when I am seeing a new breast implant patient if she will look amazing afterwards and be thrilled, or look just OK and possibly not very happy. I always tell them this honest prediction. You might say that is absurd, but I'd rather have a patient be moderately happy having told them not to expect much than one who was told they would look dynamite. By misleading patients, you will end up with a lot of unhappy people, and your reputation could be damaged.

Unfortunately, I come across patients everyday who were told by another doctor that they were a great candidate for a particular procedure, and in my estimation they certainly weren't. This is a truism in surgery: **It is much more difficult to determine who to say no to** than to do the surgery itself, and it is very hard to say no (especially when your livelihood depends on it).

Ask your potential surgeon who is a poor candidate for the procedure you're considering. It should be very easy for a doctor to describe an ideal candidate and a poor candidate for a given surgical procedure. What anatomical specifications are being considered? Everyone is not equally suitable for a procedure, but if a doctor acts that way, beware. You know that everyone is not the same. So, how can every patient be offered the same solution in some practices. For example, I know of a dermatologist who offers Coolsculpting™ non-invasive body contouring. I offer this service as well, but I don't recommend it to everyone. Some people need a tummy tuck. For others liposuction would be better. And for some, nothing at all is suggested. However, for this dermatologist, anyone who walks in the door complaining of excess fat is offered Coolsculpting™. The reason being he has no other way to treat unwanted fat. He does not know how to do surgery and therefore purchased this expensive machine so that he could enter into the realm of body contouring. So, now he must pay off this expensive equipment, and therefore everyone is offered the service. For a hammer, all the world's a nail.

4. What are the possible risks and what complications are most common?

Every surgery is required to have an accompanying surgical consent. They always list the potential risks like bleeding, infection, etc. However, that does not constitute an informed consent. An informed consent is when the surgeon himself discusses common risks and complications with the patient. **The surgeon must have an open dialogue with the patient about what might go wrong** and what would be done in that case. What are the odds for a complication? What is the worst possible outcome and what is the worst outcome he or she has actually experienced? We don't like to be negative or expect a bad outcome, but we must be realistic and actually look at the data. My nurses also review this information a second time with every patient before surgery. If there is an adverse outcome, you don't want that to be the first time the patient has ever heard of it (eg. what is a DVT?).

Here are some tough questions to ask your surgeon:

What complications do you commonly see with this procedure?

What is done to correct the complication, and *how much will that cost me?*

What is the worst complication you've ever had with this type of procedure?

Do you have some patients who I could speak with regarding their experience with your office and this procedure in particular?

Earlier I alluded to **DVT**. This stands for Deep Vein Thrombosis and is a blood clot in one of your body's major veins. The symptoms include swelling, acute pain, pain with passive movement, redness and warmth. The danger lies in the possibility that one of these blood clots would break loose from their place in the vein and travel through your inferior vena cava ultimately to the lungs. That could block oxygen exchange in your blood and lead to sudden death. This is not very common at all, but common enough that it happens to many patients every year. We take precautions to avoid DVT, such as early ambulation, intraoperative compression stockings, post-operative compression hose, and even blood thinners in high risk patients. The secret is that plastic surgeons discuss this problem a lot, amongst themselves. They only briefly touch on it with their patients. It's very scary, and many patients would potentially cancel their surgery out of fear if they were too aware of the risks. That is clearly an unethical approach. Your doctor should not skim over or totally avoid discussing uncomfortable topics. Rather, he should say here are some really bad complications, here are the frequencies with which they occur, and here is everything I do to prevent them from occurring.

5. What type of anesthesia is used and where is the procedure done?

The type of anesthesia to be used and the implications regarding that technique are important to discuss ahead of time. Even more important is who will be performing the anesthesia? Who will administer the medications and monitor the patient while he or she is asleep? Is it a nurse, a medical assistant, or the surgeon himself? Hopefully not! Although this is often the case, the best option id for either a Certified Registered Nurse Anesthetist or an Anesthesiologist (MD) to perform the anesthesia. These are professionals trained in the practice of anesthesia and not only have the experience in providing it, but will maintain complete focus on the patient's vital signs while the surgery is underway. I cannot give my complete focus to the anesthesia while I am also giving my complete focus to performing the surgery.

Finally, the setting for the surgery is very important. Without a doubt, it **must be performed in an accredited surgical facility**. This basically means in a hospital, accredited private surgery center, or accredited surgical suite within the doctor's office. Our office has two operating rooms and a recovery room. The surgical suite has been evaluated and granted accreditation with AAAASF, the AMERICAN ASSOCIATION FOR ACCREDITATION OF AMBULATORY SURGERY FACILITIES, INC. This was a tough process, and they come every so often to re-inspect our facility and verify that it is still up to par. Be very wary of a surgeon who does not have such an accreditation, or says their facility is just as good but doesn't happen to have obtained the necessary recognition. Look for accreditation by one of these organizations to ensure your surgery will be done in a safe environment: AAAASF, AAAHC, JCAHO.

Anesthesia type and provider: There are pros and cons to everything. Those who exclusively use IV sedation for their procedures tout that it is more easily tolerated, carries less post-operative nausea and vomiting, and without placing you on a ventilator is safer. Those who exclusively use general anesthesia tout that the level of anesthesia is deeper, the airway secured with a laryngeal mask or endotracheal tube, and because you are on a ventilator, it is safer. It's all in how you spin it. I think either way is acceptable. I like IV sedation because I think patients recover from the anesthetic more quickly and don't have the added risks of losing their respiratory drive during surgery, as mentioned in the previous chapter. However, I wouldn't adamantly argue that general anesthesia is unsafe. It is a viable option. What is more important, is who is performing your anesthesia and how comfortable are *they* with that particular technique.

Anesthesiologists are medical doctors who have completed a residency program (usually 3-4 years) in anesthesiology. Nurse Anesthetists (CRNAs) are usually nurses who have received a master's degree after completing a nurse anesthesia training program (2 or more years). CRNAs are usually very competent, but they are required to work under the license of a physician. When I perform surgery with a CRNA, I am the only doctor in the room. This is not a problem or a safety hazard by any means, but surgeons who happen to utilize anesthesiologists often claim their way is safer. As long as the patient understands what is going on and feels comfortable, either option is fine.

What is the setting for your surgery? Is it some sketchy hotel room near the Mexican border? I hope not! But, almost every year there is a story in the news about an unlicensed person doing plastic surgery in a hotel or motel room. Why would you ever feel comfortable meeting a "doctor" at a motel room to have a surgical procedure? I can't fathom that. It must have to do with dirt cheap prices and uneducated patients. Now, most of the time, you won't find yourself in that type of a horrific situation, but may find yourself in a nice-looking, clean surgeon's office where he plans to perform your procedure. How can a patient know if the operating room is safe? I gave you all of the most important information above. It must be accredited by one of those 3 accrediting bodies. Ask about it and ask to see a current accreditation certificate. Lots of places obtain a certificate and post their accreditation on the wall and on their website, but fail to keep it active. It takes work and quite a bit of money to renew one's credentialing every 1-2 years.

Ask for a tour of the surgical suite. We always take our pre-op patients on a tour to help them get acquainted with the facility and be more comfortable on the day of surgery. Does it look clean? Does it look modern? Do you see monitors and emergency equipment? Is there a recovery room? These are basics that even an untrained person can recognize. If you have a bad gut feeling about the environment, don't ignore that.

This is a nice, clean, appropriate modern-day operating room:

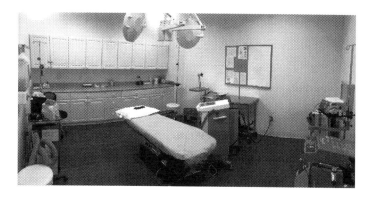

This is not:

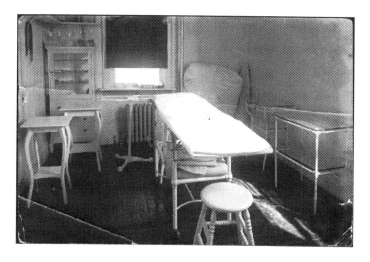

5 more secrets that are never discussed with patients:

1. **Does your surgeon operate on his or her family?**
   He shouldn't. This is considered unethical by most state
   medical boards. Are the reviews or Facebook posts by
   happy family members or unrelated patients?

2. **Fake reviews.** We work very hard for our good
   reputation. Online reviews and testimonials are hugely

important these days. Most patients read everything they can about you before ever coming in for a consultation. If the reviews are bad, or even average, they look elsewhere. Unfortunately, some disappointed patients will choose to slander you or make false allegations about their treatment being substandard. This hurts your reputation and it takes a lot of positive reviews to compensate for one negative review. In light of this, there are thousands of businesses out there, including plastic surgeons, posting fake reviews. Some sites are good at preventing it. Google is pretty good at it. Others barely make an attempt to inhibit fake reviews. Read them carefully.

Overly glowing reviews are usually (but not always) fake. Real patients say, "Dr. J was amazing and all of his staff was great to work with. I love my result and recommend him to anyone." Fake patients say, "Dr. J is without out a doubt the best plastic surgeon in the country. His technique is meticulous and his results are unbelievable. He is so kind and giving and very knowledgeable. I can't wait to have another procedure by Dr. J and tell all of my friends and family they must see him! Thank you Dr. J. I love you!!!"

3. **Not so world famous.** I come across websites every day that claim the doctor is world famous, or renowned for his technique. Really? How come I've been in practice for over 15 years and never heard of all these famous guys? Every plastic surgeon in your city can't possibly be the leading authority (except for maybe in their minds). There's nothing wrong with

being confident, but take such braggadocious claims with a grain of salt.

4. **Photoshopped pictures.** Yes, it happens. It's horrible and low. To present an altered image as an accurate representation of your work is deceiving. It happens all over the place. Magazine models are Photoshopped to look better. The food on TV commercials is altered to look better. After pictures on doctors' websites are manipulated to look better. It's hard to pick out some times, but other times it's blatantly obvious. I blur out the tattoos on my patient's pictures so that their identity is protected. That's it. I can't imagine intentionally making a picture look better than it really does to fool the public into believing I'm better than I really am. Are all of my results pure perfection? No. *I just don't show the bad pictures at all.* I have enough really good results to show without the need to Photoshop bad ones.

5. **Fake Botox.** How can doctors be using fake medications like Botox and why? These neurotoxin drugs and dermal fillers are actually quite expensive. The margin is much better if you buy dirt cheap, counterfeit alternatives. Some places say they buy their Botox from Europe, but it is still authentic Botox. I'm not sure; this may be the case. Nevertheless, it is still shady. The only drugs that should be administered in the United States are drugs purchased in the United States. Buying online or from overseas is unpredictable and of questionable safety.

I hope that this information has opened your eyes a bit to the types of information you must know before going under the knife.

All of these secrets and detailed pieces of important information are critical to understand before surgery. This is indeed a matter of life and death in some instances.

This should not scare you away from surgery, but help you choose the best surgeon and give you peace of mind that you are making the right decision. *In bocca al lupo* — good luck!

References

1. Lucy Gent and Nigel Llewellyn, eds., **Renaissance Bodies: The Human Figure in English Culture c. 1540–1660**. London: Reaktion Books, 1990.

2. Anne Ashton, Peter Humphrey, **Interpreting breast iconography in Italian art, 1250-1600**.

3. Maria Teresa Micaela Prendergast, **Renaissance Fantasies: The Gendering of Aesthetics in Early Modern Fiction**

4. Agnolo Firenzuola, Edited and translated by Konrad Eisenbichler and Jacqueline Murray, **On the Beauty of Women.** 1992

5. Jacobson, Nora, **Cleavage.** New Brunswick: Rutgers. p. 48, 2000.

6. Bondurant S, Ernster V, Herdman R (eds); Committee on the Safety of Silicone Breast Implants, **Safety of Silicone Breast Implants.** Institute of Medicine. p. 21, 1990.

7. Hester TR Jr, Tebbetts JB, Maxwell GP, **The Polyurethane-covered Mammary Prosthesis: Facts and Fiction (II): A Look Back and a "peek" Ahead**, Clinical Plastic Surgery **28** (3): 579–86, 2001.

8. http://psychcentral.com/news/2007/03/23/plastic-surgery-helps-self-esteem/703.html

9. Kelly HA, **Report of gynecological cases (excessive growth of fat)**. *Johns Hopkins Med J.* 1899; 10:197.

10. Kelly HA, **Excision of fat of the abdominal wall lipectomy.** *Surg Gynecol Obstet.* 1910; 10:229.

11. Thorek M., **Plastic Surgery of the Breast and Abdominal Wall,** Springfield, Ill: Thomas; 1924.

12. Thorek M., **Plastic reconstruction of the female breast and abdomen.** *Am J Surg.* 1939; 43:268.

13. Pitanguy I., **Abdominolipectomy. An approach to it through an analysis of 300 consecutive cases.** *Plast Reconstr Surg.* 1967; 40:384.

14. Regnault P., **Abdominal lipectomy, a low "W" incision.** New York International Society of Aesthetic Plastic Surgery; 1972.

15. Grazer FM., **Abdominoplasty.** *Plast Reconstr Surg.* Jun 1973; 51(6):617-23.

16. Charles Conrad Miller, **Cosmetic surgery : the correction of featural imperfections;** 1908.

Printed in the United States
By Bookmasters